CW00468299

The Ultimate
Keto Diet For Women
Over 50

Quick, Easy and Healthy Recipes for
Busy People on Keto Diet

Tiffany Johnson

TABLE OF CONTENTS

INTRODUCTION

Y ou all know that our body needs energy for its functioning and the energy sources come from carbohydrates, proteins, and fats. Owing to years of conditioning that a low-fat carbohydrate-rich diet is essential for good health, we have become used to depending on glucose (from carbohydrates) to get most of the energy that our body needs. Only when the amount of glucose available for energy generation decreases, does our body begin to break down fat for drawing energy to power our cells and organs. This is the express purpose of a ketogenic diet.

The primary aim of a ketogenic diet (called simply as keto diet) is to convert your body into a fat-burning machine. Such a diet is loaded with benefits and is highly recommended by nutritional experts for the following end results:

- Natural appetite control
- Increased mental clarity
- Lowered levels of inflammation in the body system
- Improved stability in blood sugar levels
- Elimination or lower risk of heartburn
- Using natural stored body fat as the fuel source
- Weight loss

The effects listed are just some of the numerous effects that take place when a person embarks on a ketogenic diet and makes it a point to stick to it. A ketogenic diet consists of meals with low carbohydrates, moderate proteins, and high-fat content. The mechanism works like this: when we drastically reduce the intake of carbohydrates, our body is compelled to convert fat for releasing energy. This process of converting fats instead of carbohydrates to release energy is called ketosis.

Health Benefits of Keto Diet to Women Above 50

Both low-fat and also low-carb diet plans can be reliable for weight loss, according to the American Association of Retired Persons (AARP). The low-carb diet has some extra health and wellness advantages worth taking into consideration. The researcher also went so far as to recommend that the low-carb diet plan might provide a choice to pain-relieving opioids.

In addition, low-carb diet plans might aid HDL (good) cholesterol and triglyceride degrees much more efficiently than even more carb-heavy diet plans,

According to the Mayo Clinic. Today, low-carb diet plans have taken a number of popular types, consisting of the keto diet plan, the paleo diet plan and the Mediterranean diet. While each of these choices includes its own nuances, they're all based around lowering carbohydrate intake, while raising healthy and balanced fat consumption.

Decreased Thyroid Function

Research study has discovered that a ketogenic diet plan lowers the degree of T3, the body's active thyroid hormonal agent. Unfortunately, this suggests a ketogenic diet might not be optimal for those with preexisting hypothyroidism. Consult with your physician first since you may require thyroid assistance if you have hypothyroidism and also want to continue with a ketogenic diet plan.

Elevated Cortisol

Research study has suggested that a ketogenic diet plan raises the tension hormonal agent cortisol to increase power levels despite reduced carbohydrate availability. It is still up for debate whether this increase in cortisol is innocuous or dangerous. Getting a lot of rest, exercising, and engaging in a routine stress-reduction technique can assist you to keep your standard tension degrees reduced and decrease the possibility for consistently elevated cortisol.

Nutrient deficiencies: Older grownups often tend to have more significant shortages in essential nutrients like:

Iron: the deficiency can lead to mental fog and also exhaustion

Vitamin B12: deficiency can cause neurological problems like dementia.

Fats: deficiency can lead to troubles with cognition, vitamin, vision, and even skin shortages.

Vitamin D: deficiency can cause cognitive problems in older grownups, raise the danger of cardiovascular disease and also contribute to cancer cells threat. The top-quality resources of animal protein on the ketogenic diet plan can quickly account for excellent sources of these essential nutrients.

Regulating Blood Sugar

As we've talked about, the connection between poor blood sugar and also brain associated circumstances like Alzheimer's disease, mental weakening, and Parkinson's disease exists. Excess consumption of carbohydrates, mainly from fructose, which is drastically lowered in the ketogenic diet

An absence of nutritional fats and cholesterol-- which are bountiful and also healthy and balanced on the ketogenic diet plan.

Oxidative stress and anxiety, which being in ketosis prevents. Making use of a ketogenic diet to assist in regulating blood sugar levels and improve nourishment might assist not only improve insulin response, but also secure against memory issues that frequently transpire with age.

Keto foods provide a high amount of nutrition per calorie. This is crucial because basal metabolic rate (the number of calories needed daily to endure) is less for seniors, yet they still need the same quantity of nutrients as younger people.

A person age 50+ will have a much more challenging time residing on junk foods than a teenager or 20+ whose body is still resilient. This makes it also a lot more important for seniors to eat foods that are disease fighting and health-supporting. It can necessarily imply the difference between enjoying the golden years to the max and spending them suffering and in pain.

Elderly women need to consume a much more optimal diet plan by avoiding "vacant calories" from sugars or foods rich in anti-nutrients, such as whole grains and also increasing their amount of nutrient-rich fats and healthy proteins.

Additionally, much of the food chosen by older people (or given up medical facility or clinical settings) often tend to be significantly refined and very poor in nutrients, such as white bread, pasta, prunes, mashed potatoes, puddings, and so on.

It's quite clear that the high-carb diet so commonly pushed by the government is not best for sustaining our senior women and also their lasting health and wellness. A diet plan low in carbs and abundant in animal and plant fats is much better for advertising much better insulin level of sensitivity, and also overall better health and wellness.

Ketosis for Longevity

No matter our age, it's never a bad idea to improve your possibilities of sensation and also to operate well for the remainder of your life. It's never far too late to begin doing better, even though the faster we begin, the better our opportunities for avoiding the condition. Also, for those that have invested lots of years not treating their bodies as they should, ketosis for senior citizens has the potential to repair a few of the damage.

That being stated, the earlier we can start making changes that support healthy and balanced weight, blood sugar, immunity, and extra, the greater the chance of having less pain and suffering later on in life. Note: We're all growing older, and death is, naturally, unavoidable. What we can control to a degree is the top quality of a lasting life with the keto method.

People are currently living much longer; however, we're additionally getting sicker by complying with the typical diet plan of the majority. The ketogenic diet can help elders boost their wellness, so they can grow, instead of being ill or hurting during the later years of life.

Because your body turns fat from your diet plan and your inner fat shops into ketones, the keto diet rapidly enhances weight loss. And also, unlike sugar, ketones cannot be stored as fat since they aren't digested similarly.

That's surprising? For decades, you've heard that fat makes you add weight. Your body is developed to make use of fat as a different resource of energy. For the majority of background, people weren't consuming three-square meals and snacks throughout the day.

BREAKFAST

1. Smoky Pork with Cabbage

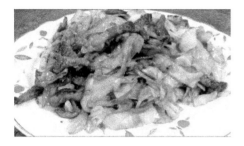

Preparation Time: 10 minutes

Cooking Time: 8 hours

Servings: 6

Ingredients:

- 3 lbs. pastured pork roast
- 1/3 cup liquid smoke
- 1/2 cabbage head, chopped
- 1 cup water
- 1 tbsp... kosher salt

Directions:

1. Rub pork with kosher salt and place into the slow cooker.
2. Pour liquid smoke over the pork. Add water.
3. Cover and cook on low.

4. Remove pork from slow cooker and add cabbage in the bottom of slow cooker.

5. Now place pork on top of the cabbage.

6. Cover again and cook.

7. Shred pork with a fork and serve.

Nutrition: Calories 484 Fat 21.5 g Carbs 3.5 g Sugar 1.9 g Protein 65.4 g Cholesterol 195 mg

2. Italian Frittata

Preparation Time: 10 minutes

Cooking Time: 4 hours

Servings: 4

Ingredients:

- 6 eggs
- 1/4 cup cherry tomatoes, sliced
- 4 oz... mushrooms, sliced
- 2 tsp.... Italian seasoning
- 1/2 cup cheddar cheese, shredded
- Pepper
- Salt

Directions:

1. Add mushrooms and cherry tomatoes to the pan and cook until softened.
2. Transfer vegetables to the crock pot.
3. In a bowl, whisk together eggs, cheese, pepper, and salt.
4. Pour egg mixture in the crock pot.
5. Cover and cook on low.
6. Slice and serve.

Nutrition: Calories 167 Fat 12 g Carbs 2.3 g Sugar 1.6 g Protein 12.8 g Cholesterol 262 mg

3. Cauliflower Casserole

Preparation Time: 10 minutes

Cooking Time: 6 hours

Servings: 8

Ingredients:

- 12 eggs
- 1/2 cup unsweetened almond milk
- 1 lb. sausage, cooked and crumbled
- 1 cauliflower head, shredded
- 2 cups cheddar cheese, shredded
- Pepper
- Salt

Directions:

1. Spray a crock pot inside with cooking spray.
2. Combine together eggs, almond milk, pepper, and salt.
3. Add about a third of the shredded cauliflower into the bottom of the crock pot. Season with pepper and salt.
4. Pour egg mixture into the crock pot.
5. Cover and cook on low
6. Serve and enjoy.

Nutrition: Calories 443 Fat 35.6 g Carbs 3.5 g Sugar 2 g Protein 27.4 g Cholesterol 323 mg

4. Balsamic Chicken

Preparation Time: 10 minutes

Cooking Time: 3 hours

Servings: 8

Ingredients:

- 3 lb. chicken breasts, sliced in half
- 3/4 cup balsamic vinegar
- 2 tsp.... dried onion, minced
- 2 tsp.... dried basil
- 3 garlic cloves, minced
- 1 Tbsp... olive oil
- 1/4 tsp.... pepper
- 1/2 tsp.... salt

Directions:

1. Add garlic and olive oil to a crock pot.
2. In a small bowl, mix together the dry seasonings.
3. Rub chicken breasts with the seasonings and place them in the crock pot.
4. Pour balsamic vinegar over chicken breasts.
5. Cover and cook on low.
6. Slice and serve.

Nutrition: Calories 345 Fat 14.4 g Carbs 0.7 g Sugar 0.1 g Protein 49.3 g Cholesterol 151 mg

5. Easy Mexican Chicken

Preparation Time: 10 minutes

Cooking Time: 5 hours

Servings: 4

Ingredients:

- 8 chicken thighs, -
- 1/4 tsp. red pepper
- 1/4 cup onion,
- 1 packet taco
- 1 cup chicken stock

Directions:

1. Combine stock to a crock pot. Stir well to blend.
2. Spread remaining seasoning on top of chicken.
3. Cover and cook on low
4. Brush with red pepper flakes and green onions.
5. Enjoy!

Nutrition: Calories 565 Fat 21.8 g Carbs 1.7 g Sugar 0.6 g Protein 84.8 g Cholesterol 260 mg

LUNCH

6. Chicken Fajitas

Preparation Time: 10 minutes

Cooking Time: 3 hours

Servings: 6

Ingredients:

- 11/2 lb. chicken breast fillet
- 1/2cup salsa
- 2oz. cream cheese
- 1teaspoon cumin
- 1teaspoon paprika
- Salt and pepper to taste
- 1onion, sliced
- 1clove garlic, minced
- 1red bell pepper, sliced
- 1green bell pepper, sliced
- 1teaspoon lime juice

Directions:

1. Combine all the ingredients except the lime wedges in your slow cooker.
2. Cover the pot.
3. Cook on high for 3 hours.

4. Shred the chicken.

5. Drizzle with lime juice.

6. Serve with toppings like sour cream and cheese.

Nutrition: Calories 276 Fat 17 g Cholesterol 105 mg Sodium 827 mg Carbohydrate 3 g Protein 25 g Sugars 2 g

7. Tuscan Garlic Chicken

Preparation Time: 15 minutes

Cooking Time: 3 hours

Servings: 6

Ingredients:

- 1tablespoon olive oil
- 2cloves garlic, crushed and minced
- 1/2cup chicken broth
- 1cup heavy cream
- 3/4cup Parmesan cheese, grated
- 2chicken breasts
- 1tablespoon Italian seasoning
- Salt and pepper to taste
- 1/2 cup sundried tomatoes, chopped
- 2 cups spinach, chopped

Directions:

1. Pour the oil into your pan over medium heat.
2. Cook the garlic for 1 minute.
3. Stir in the broth and cream.
4. Simmer for 10 minutes.
5. Stir in the Parmesan cheese and remove from heat.
6. Put the chicken in your slow cooker.
7. Season with the salt, pepper and Italian seasoning.

8. Place the tomatoes on top of the chicken.

9. Pour the cream mixture on top of the chicken.

10. Cover the pot.

11. Cook on high for 3 hours.

12. Take the chicken out of the slow cooker and set aside

13. Add the spinach and stir until wilted.

14. Pour the sauce over the chicken and serve with the sun-dried tomatoes and spinach.

Nutrition: Calories 306 Fat 18.4g Cholesterol 115mg Sodium 287mg Carbohydrate 4.9g Protein 30.1g Sugars 2g Sugars 2 g

8. Ranch Chicken

Preparation Time: 5 minutes

Cooking Time: 4 hours and 5 minutes

Servings: 6

Ingredients:

- 2lb. chicken breast fillet
- 2tablespoons butter
- 2oz. cream cheese
- 3tablespoons ranch dressing mix

Directions:

1. Add the chicken to your slow cooker.
2. Place the butter and cream cheese on top of the chicken.
3. Sprinkle ranch dressing mix.
4. Seal the pot.
5. Cook on high for 4 hours.
6. Shred the chicken using forks and serve.

Nutrition: Calories 266 Fat 12.9 g Sodium 167 mg Potassium 450 mg Carbohydrate 4 g Fiber 0 g Protein 33 g Sugars 3 g

9. Chicken with Green Beans

Preparation Time: 5 minutes

Cooking Time: 4 hours

Servings: 4

Ingredients:

- 1onion, diced
- 2cloves garlic, crushed and minced
- 2tomatoes, diced
- 1/4cup dill, chopped
- 1lb. green beans
- 1cup chicken broth
- 1tablespoon lemon juice
- 6chicken thighs
- Salt and pepper to taste
- 2tablespoons olive oil

Directions:

1. Put the onion, garlic, tomatoes, dill and green beans in your slow cooker.
2. Pour in the chicken broth and lemon juice.
3. Season with salt and pepper.
4. Mix well.
5. Add the chicken on top of the vegetables
6. Drizzle chicken with oil.

7. Cover the pot.

8. Cook on high for 4 hours.

Nutrition: Calories 373 Fat 26 g Sodium 315 mg Carbohydrate 1.4 g Fiber 4 g Protein 22 g Sugars 6 g

10. Greek Chicken

Preparation Time: 15 minutes

Cooking Time: 2 hours

Servings: 6

Ingredients:

- 2tablespoons olive oil
- 2cloves garlic
- 2lb. chicken thigh fillets
- Salt and pepper to taste
- 1cup calamite olives
- 2oz. marinated artichoke hearts, rinsed and drained
- 3oz. roasted red peppers, drained and sliced
- 1onion, sliced
- 1/2cup chicken broth
- 1/4cup red wine vinegar
- 1tablespoon lemon juice
- 1teaspoon dried oregano
- 1teaspoon dried thyme
- 2tablespoons arrowroot starch

Directions:

1. Season the chicken with salt and pepper.
2. Put a pan over medium high heat.
3. Add the oil and garlic.

4. Cook for 1 minute, stirring frequently.

5. Add the chicken and cook for 2 minutes per side.

6. Transfer the chicken to the slow cooker.

7. Add the olives, artichoke hearts and peppers around the chicken.

8. Sprinkle onion on top.

9. In a bowl, mix the rest of the ingredients except the arrowroot starch.

10. Pour this into the slow cooker.

11. Cover the pot.

12. Cook on high for 2 hours.

13. Get 3 tablespoons of the cooking liquid.

14. Stir in the arrowroot starch to the liquid and put it back to the pot.

15. Simmer for 15 minutes before serving.

Nutrition: Calories 452 Fat 36 g Sodium 899 mg Carbohydrate 4 g Fiber 1 g Protein 26 g Sugars 3 g

11. Shrimp Scampi

Preparation Time: 15 minutes

Cooking Time: 3 hours

Servings: 4

Ingredients:

- 1/4cup chicken bone broth
- 1/2cup white cooking wine
- 2tablespoons olive oil
- 2tablespoons butter
- 1tablespoon garlic, minced
- 2tablespoons parsley, chopped
- 1tablespoon lemon juice
- Salt and pepper to taste
- 1lb. shrimp, peeled and deveined

Directions:

1. Mix all the ingredients in your slow cooker.
2. Cover the pot.
3. Cook on low for 3 hours.

Nutrition: Calories 256 Fat 14.7 g Sodium 466 mg Carbohydrate 2.1 g Fiber 0.1 g Protein 23.3 g Sugars 2 g

12. **<u>Shrimp Boil</u>**

Preparation Time: 15 minutes

Cooking Time: 4 hours

Servings: 4

Ingredients:

- 11/2 lb. potatoes, sliced into wedges
- 2cloves garlic, peeled
- 2ears corn
- 1lb. sausage, sliced
- 1/4cup Old Bay seasoning
- 1tablespoon lemon juice
- 2cups water
- 2lb. shrimp, peeled

Directions:

1. Put the potatoes in your slow cooker. Add the garlic, corn and sausage in layers.
2. Season with the Old Bay seasoning.
3. Drizzle lemon juice on top.
4. Pour in the water.
5. Do not mix.
6. Cover the pot.
7. Cook on high for 4 hours.
8. Add the shrimp on top.

9. Cook for 15 minutes.

Nutrition: Calories 585 Fat 25.1g Sodium 2242mg Potassium 1166mg Carbohydrate 3.7g Fiber 4.9g Protein 53.8g Sugars 3.9g

13. Shrimp & Sausage Gumbo

Preparation Time: 15 minutes

Cooking Time: 1 hour and 15 minutes

Servings: 4

Ingredients:

- 2tablespoons olive oil
- 2lb. chicken thigh fillet, sliced into cubes
- 2cloves garlic, crushed and minced
- 1onion, sliced
- 2stalks celery, chopped
- 1green bell pepper, chopped
- 1teaspoon Cajun seasoning
- Salt to taste
- 2cups beef broth
- 28oz. canned crushed tomatoes
- 4oz. sausage
- 2tablespoons butter
- 1lb. shrimp, peeled and deveined

Directions:

1. Pour the olive oil in a pan over medium heat.
2. Cook the garlic and chicken for 5 minutes.
3. Add the onion, celery and bell pepper.
4. Cook until tender.

5. Season with the Cajun seasoning and salt.

6. Cook for 2 minutes.

7. Stir in the sausage, broth and tomatoes.

8. Cover and cook on low for 1 hour.

9. Add the butter and shrimp in the last 10 minutes of cooking.

Nutrition: Calories 467 Fat 33 g Sodium 1274 mg Potassium 658 mg Carbohydrate 5 g Fiber 2 g Protein 33 g Sugars 5 g

14. Fish Stew

Preparation Time: 15 minutes

Cooking Time: 1 hour and 24 minutes

Servings: 2

Ingredients

- 1lb. white fish
- 1tablespoon lime juice
- 1onion, sliced
- 2cloves garlic, sliced
- 1red pepper, sliced
- 1jalapeno pepper, sliced
- 1teaspoon paprika
- 2cups chicken broth
- 2cups tomatoes, chopped
- Salt and pepper to taste
- 2oz. coconut milk

Directions:

1. Marinate the fish in lime juice for 10 minutes.
2. Pour the olive oil into a pan over medium heat.
3. Add the onion, garlic and peppers.
4. Cook for 4 minutes.
5. Add the rest of the ingredients except the coconut milk.
6. Cover the pot.

7. Cook on low for 1 hour.

8. Stir in the coconut milk and simmer for 10 minutes

Nutrition: Calories 323 Fat 28.6g Sodium 490mg Carbohydrate 1.1g Protein 9.3g Fiber 3.2g Sugars 6.2g

DINNER

15. Ragu

Preparation Time: 10 minutes

Cooking Time: 8 hours

Servings: 2

Ingredients:

- 1/4Carrot
- 1/4Rib of celery
- 1/4Onion
- 1/41 minced garlic clove
- 1/2 lb. top-round lean beef
- 3oz.Diced tomatoes
- 3oz.Crushed tomatoes
- 2tsp. beef broth
- 11/4tsp.Chopped fresh thyme
- 11/4tsp.Minced fresh rosemary
- 1bay leaf
- Pepper & Salt to taste

Directions:

1. Place the prepared celery, garlic, onion, and carrots into the slow cooker.

2. Trim away the fat, and add the meat to the slow cooker. Sprinkle with the salt and pepper

3. Stir in the rest of the ingredients.

4. Prepare on the low setting for six to eight hours. Enjoy any way you choose.

Nutrition: Calories: 224 Carbs: 5 g Protein: 27 g Fat: 9 g

16. Rope Vieja

Preparation Time: 15 minutes

Cooking Time: 8 hours

Servings: 6

Ingredients:

- 2 lb. flank steak – remove fat
- 1tsp.Yellow pepper
- 1Thinly sliced onion
- 1Green pepper
- 1Bay leaf
- 1/4tsp. salt
- 3/4Oregano
- 3/4-fat beef broth
- 3/41 tbsp. tomato paste
- Cooking spray

Directions:

1. Prepare the crockpot with the spray or use a liner and combine all of the fixings.
2. Stir everything together and prepare using low for eight hours.
3. Top it off with your chosen garnishes.

Nutrition: Calories: 257 Carbs: 4 g Fat: 10 g Protein: 35 g

17. Spinach Soup

Preparation Time: 15 minutes

Cooking Time: 6-8 hours

Servings: 4

Ingredients:

- 2 pounds' spinach
- 1/4 cup cream cheese
- 1 onion, diced
- 2 cups heavy cream
- 1 garlic clove, minced
- 2 cups water
- salt, pepper, to taste

Directions:

1. Pour water into the slow cooker. Add spinach, salt, and pepper.
2. Add cream cheese, onion, garlic, and heavy cream.
3. Close the lid and cook on Low for 6-8 hours.
4. Puree soup with blender and serve.

Nutrition: Calories: 322 Fats: 28.2g Carbs: 1.1g Protein: 12.2g

18. Mashed Cauliflower with Herbs

Preparation Time: 15 minutes

Cooking Time: 3-6 hours

Servings: 4

Ingredients:

- 1 cauliflower head, cut into florets
- 3 garlic cloves, peeled
- 1/2 teaspoon fresh rosemary, chopped
- 1/2 teaspoon fresh thyme, chopped
- 1/2 teaspoon fresh sage, chopped
- 1/2 teaspoon fresh parsley, chopped
- 1 cup vegetable broth
- 2 cups water
- 2 tablespoons, ghee
- Salt, pepper, to taste

Directions:

1. Pour broth into the slow cooker, add cauliflower florets.
2. Add water, it should cover the cauliflower.
3. Close the lid and cook on Low for 6 hours or on High for 3 hours.
4. Once cooked, drain water from the slow cooker.
5. Add herbs, salt, pepper, and ghee, puree with a blender.

Nutrition: Calories 115 Fats 12g carbs 4.7g Protein 6.2g

19. Kale Quiche

Preparation Time: 15 minutes

Cooking Time: 3-5 hours

Servings: 3

Ingredients:

- 1 cup almond milk
- 2 eggs
- 1 cup Carb Quick Baking Mix
- 2 cups spinach, chopped
- 1/2 bell pepper, chopped
- 2 cups fresh baby kale, chopped
- 1 teaspoon garlic, chopped
- 1/3 cup fresh basil, chopped
- Salt, pepper, to taste
- 1 tablespoon olive oil

Directions:

1. Add oil to a slow cooker or use a cooking spray.
2. Beat eggs into a slow cooker; add almond milk and Baking Mix, mix to combine.
3. Add spinach, bell pepper, garlic, and basil, stir to combine.
4. Close the lid and cook on Low for 5 hours or on High for 3 hours.
5. Make sure the quiche is done, check the center with a toothpick, it should be dry.

Nutrition: Calories: 273 Fats: 24.4g Carbs: 5.g Protein: 10.5g

20. Spinach Stuffed Portobello

Preparation Time: 15 minutes

Cooking Time: 3 hours

Servings: 8

Ingredients:

- 2 oz. medium-sized Portobello mushrooms, stems removed
- 2 tablespoons olive oil
- 1/2 onion, chopped
- 2 cups fresh spinach, rinsed and chopped
- 3 garlic cloves, minced
- 1 cup chicken broth
- 3 tablespoons parmesan cheese, grated
- 1/3 teaspoon dried thyme
- Salt, pepper, to taste

Directions:

1. Heat oil in a medium pan over high heat.

2. Add onion, cook until translucent, stirring steadily. Add spinach and thyme, cook for 1-2 minutes until spinach is wilted.

3. Brush each mushroom with olive oil.

4. Put 1 tablespoon of onion and spinach stuffing into each mushroom.

5. Pour chicken broth into the slow cooker. Put stuffed mushrooms on the bottom.

6. Close the lid and cook on High for 3 hours.

7. Once cooked, sprinkle mushrooms with parmesan cheese and serve.

Nutrition: Calories 310g Fats 21g Carbs 3g Protein 12g

21. Cod and Vegetables

Preparation Time: 15 minutes

Cooking Time: 1-3 hours

Servings: 4

Ingredients:

- 5-6 oz. cod fillets
- 1 bell pepper, sliced or chopped
- 1 onion, sliced
- 1/2 fresh lemon, sliced
- 1 zucchini, sliced
- 3 garlic cloves, minced
- 1/4 cup low-sodium broth
- 1 teaspoon rosemary
- 1/4 teaspoon red pepper flakes
- Salt, pepper, to taste

Directions:

1. Season cod fillets with salt and pepper.
2. Pour broth into a slow cooker, add garlic, rosemary, bell pepper, onion, and zucchini into the slow cooker.
3. Put fish into your crockpot, add lemon slices on top.
4. Close the lid and cook on Low for 2-3 hours or on High for 1 hour.

Nutrition: Calories 150 Fats 11.6g Carbs 2g Protein 26.9g

22. Ribeye with Caramelized Onions and Mushrooms

Preparation Time: 15 minutes

Cooking Time: 15 minutes

Servings: 10

Ingredients:

- 2 (6-ounce) ribeye steaks
- 1tablespoon olive oil
- Salt
- Freshly ground black pepper
- 1/2tablespoons ghee or salted butter
- 1 yellow onion, sliced
- 1 cup sliced mushrooms

Directions:

1. Pat the steaks dry with paper towels, then rub them with the olive oil. Season generously with salt and pepper.

2. In a large skillet over medium heat, heat the butter. Add the onion and cook, stirring frequently, for 3 to 5 minutes, until it starts to soften. Add the mushrooms and cook until the mushrooms are tender and the onion is translucent, another 5 minutes or so. Transfer the mixture to a paper towel–lined plate.

3. In the skillet over medium-high heat, grill the steak for 4 to 5 minutes on each side, to your desired doneness. Plate the steaks and let rest for 5 minutes.

4. Serve the steak immediately with the mushrooms and onion spooned over the top.

Nutrition: Calories: 519; Protein: 52g; Carbs: 5g; Fiber: 1g;

23. Beef Stroganoff

Preparation Time: 5 minutes

Cooking Time: 20 minutes

Servings: 2

Ingredients:

- 1pound ground beef
- 1 tablespoon salted butter
- 1 yellow onion, diced
- 2cups mushrooms, sliced
- 1garlic cloves, minced
- 1 cup beef broth
- 1 cup sour cream
- 1/4 teaspoon xanthan gum
- Salt
- Freshly ground black pepper
- Chopped fresh parsley, for garnish (optional)
- Grated Parmesan cheese, for garnish (optional)

Directions:

1. . In a large skillet over medium-high heat, cook the ground beef, stirring and breaking it up with a spatula, until cooked through, 7 to 10 minutes. Drain the fat and transfer the meat to a paper towel–lined plate.

2. In the same skillet still over medium-high heat, melt the butter. Add the onion, mushrooms, and garlic and cook, stirring frequently, until the garlic is browned and the onion and mushrooms are tender, 5 to 7 minutes.

3. Add the broth, browned beef, sour cream, and xanthan gum to the skillet and cook, stirring, until the sauce is combined and thickened, 3 to 5 minutes.

4. Serve hot, garnished with the fresh parsley and grated Parmesan cheese (if using).

Directions: Calories: 369; Total Fat: 25g; Protein: 28g; Carbs: 5g;

24. Flank Steak and Broccoli

Preparation Time: 10 minutes

Cooking Time: 30 minutes

Servings: 4

Ingredients:

- 1pound flank steak
- 6 tablespoons olive oil, divided
- 1 teaspoon garlic powder
- 1 teaspoon onion powder
- Salt
- Freshly ground black pepper
- 4 cups broccoli florets

Directions:

1. In a large, resealable plastic bag, combine the steak and 3 tablespoons of olive oil with the garlic powder and onion powder. Season with salt and pepper. Refrigerate for at least 30 minutes, or up to 24 hours.

2. Set the oven broiler to high. Line a sheet pan with aluminum foil.

3. Place the steak and broccoli on the prepared sheet pan. Drizzle the remaining 3 tablespoons of olive oil over the broccoli, and season with salt and pepper. Toss until coated.

4. Cook under the broiler for 3 to 5 minutes, then flip the steak and continue to cook for 3 to 5 minutes more, or until the steak reaches your preferred doneness.

5. Let the steak rest for 10 minutes, then slice it thinly across the grain and serve with the roasted broccoli on the side.

Nutrition: Calories: 380; Fat: 30g; Protein: 26g; Carbs: 5g;

25. Barbecue Spare Ribs

Preparation Time: 15 minutes

Cooking Time: 5 hrs.

Servings: 5

Ingredients:

- 2 pounds' spare ribs
- 1/2tablespoon salt
- 1 tablespoon garlic powder
- 1 tablespoon onion powder
- 1 tablespoon paprika
- 1 teaspoon ground cumin
- 1 teaspoon freshly ground black pepper

Directions:

1. Pat the ribs dry with paper towels, and slice them into sections to fit in the slow cooker.

2. In a small bowl, stir together the salt, garlic powder, onion powder, paprika, cumin, and pepper. Rub the seasoning mixture all over the ribs.

3. Place the ribs in the slow cooker and cook on low for 8 to 10 hours or on high for 4 to 5 hours, until the meat is very tender and falling off the bones.

4. Serve hot.

Nutrition: Calories: 263g; Fat: 19g; Protein: 21g; Carbs: 1g; Fiber: 0g

26. Slow Cooker Pork Chili Colorado

Preparation Time: 10 minutes

Cooking Time: 8 hrs.

Servings: 8

Ingredients:

- 2 pounds' boneless pork shoulder, cut into 1-inch cubes
- 1onion, chopped
- 1/2tablespoons chili powder
- 1 tablespoon chipotle chili powder
- 1 teaspoon sea salt
- Juice of 1 lime
- 1 avocado, cubed
- 1/2 cup grated Monterey Jack cheese
- 1/2 cup sour cream
- 1/4 cup chopped, fresh cilantro
- 6 green onions, sliced

Directions:

1. In a slow cooker, combine the pork shoulder, onion, chili powder, chipotle, and salt. Cover and cook on low for eight to ten hours, until the pork is soft.

2. Stir in the lime juice.

3. Serve garnished with the avocado, cheese, sour cream, cilantro, and onion.

Nutrition: Calories: 451; Fat: 33g Protein: 32g; Carbs: 5g; Fiber: 3g;

27. Thyme Sea Bass

Preparation Time: 15 minutes

Cooking Time: 15 minutes

Servings: 10

Ingredients:

- 11 oz. sea bass, trimmed
- 2 tablespoons coconut cream
- 3 oz. spring onions, chopped
- 1 teaspoon fennel seeds
- 1/2 teaspoon dried thyme
- 1 teaspoon olive oil
- 1/3 cup water
- 1 teaspoon apple cider vinegar
- 1/2 teaspoon salt

Directions:

1. In the slow cooker, mix the sea bass with the cream and the other ingredients.
2. Close the lid and cook sea bass for 4 hours on Low.

Nutrition: Calories 304, Fat 11.4, Fiber 0.9, Carbs 2.6, Protein 0.7

28. **Butter-dipped Lobsters**

Preparation Time: 15 minutes

Cooking Time: 1 hour

Servings: 3

Ingredients:

- 4 lb. lobster tails, cut in half
- 4 tablespoons of unsalted butter, melted
- Salt to taste
- Black pepper to taste

Directions:

1. Start by throwing all the Ingredients: into your Crockpot.
2. Cover its lid and cook for 1 hour on Low setting.
3. Once done, remove its lid and give it a stir.
4. Serve warm.

Nutrition: Calories 324 Fat 20.7 g Carbs 3.6 g Sugar 1.4 g Fiber 0.5 g Protein 15.3 g

SNACKS RECIPES

29. Cauliflower Poppers

Preparation Time: 20 minutes

Cooking Time: 30 minutes

Servings: 4

Ingredients:

- 4 C. cauliflower florets
- 2 tsp. olive oil
- 1/4 tsp. chili powder
- Pepper and salt

Directions:

1. Preheat the oven to 4500 F. Grease a roasting pan.
2. In a bowl, add all ingredients and toss to coat well.
3. Transfer the cauliflower mixture into a prepared roasting pan and spread in an even layer.
4. Roast for about 25-30 minutes.
5. Serve warm.

Nutrition: Calories: 102 Fat: 8.5g Fiber: 4.7g Carbohydrates: 2.1 g Protein: 4.2g

30. Crispy Parmesan Chips

Preparation Time: 10 minutes

Cooking Time: 5 minutes

Servings: 8

Ingredients:

- 1 teaspoon butter
- 8 ounces full-fat Parmesan cheese, shredded or freshly grated

Directions:

1. Preheat the oven to 400°F.
2. The Parmesan cheese must be spooned onto the baking sheet in mounds, spread evenly apart.
3. Spread out the mounds with the back of a spoon until they are flat.
4. Bake the crackers until the edges are browned, and the centers are still pale about 5 minutes.

Nutrition: Calories: 101 Fat: 9.4g Fiber: 3.1g Carbohydrates: 2.5 g Protein: 1.2g

31. Tex-Mex Queso Dip

Preparation Time: 5 minutes

Cooking Time: 10 minutes

Servings: 6

Ingredients:

- 1/2 cup of coconut milk
- 1/2 jalapeño pepper, seeded and diced
- 1teaspoon minced garlic
- 1/2 teaspoon onion powder
- 1ounces goat cheese
- 6 ounces sharp Cheddar cheese, shredded
- 1/4 teaspoon cayenne pepper

Directions:

1. Preheat a pot then add the coconut milk, jalapeño, garlic, and onion powder.
2. Simmer then whisk in the goat cheese until smooth.
3. Add the Cheddar cheese and cayenne and whisk until the dip is thick, 30 seconds to 1 minute.

Nutrition: Calories: 149 Fat: 12.1g Fiber: 3.1g Carbohydrates: 5.1 g Protein: 4.2g

32. Sweet Onion Dip

Preparation Time: 15 minutes

Cooking Time: 25-30 minutes

Servings: 4

Ingredients:

- 3 cup sweet onion chopped
- tsp. pepper sauce
- cups Swiss cheese shredded
- Ground black pepper
- cups mayonnaise
- 1/4 cup horseradish

Directions:

1. Take a bowl, add sweet onion, horseradish, pepper sauce, mayonnaise, and Swiss cheese, mix them well and transfer into the pie plate.

2. Preheat oven at 375.

3. Now put the plate into the oven and bake for 25 to 30 minutes until edges turn golden brown.

4. Sprinkle pepper to taste and serve with crackers.

Nutrition: Calories: 278 Fat: 11.4g Fiber: 4.1g Carbohydrates: 2.9 g Protein: 6.9g

33. Keto Trail Mix

Preparation Time: 5 minutes

Cooking Time: 0 minutes

Servings: 3

Ingredients:

- 1/2 cup salted pumpkin seeds

- 1/2 cup slivered almonds

- 3/4 cup roasted pecan halves

- 3/4 cup unsweetened cranberries

- 1cup toasted coconut flakes

Directions:

1. In a skillet, place almonds and pecans. Heat for 2-3 minutes and let cool.

2. Once cooled, in a large resealable plastic bag, combine all ingredients.

3. Seal and shake vigorously to mix.

4. Evenly divide into suggested Servings: and store in airtight meal prep containers.

Nutrition: Calories: 98 Fat: 1.2g Fiber: 4.1g Carbohydrates: 1.1 g Protein: 3.2g

34. Cold Cuts and Cheese Pinwheels

Preparation Time: 20 minutes

Cooking Time: 0 minutes

Servings: 2

Ingredients:

- 8 ounces' cream cheese, at room temperature
- 1/4-pound salami, thinly sliced
- 2 tablespoons sliced pepperoncini

Directions:

1. Layout a sheet of plastic wrap on a large cutting board or counter.

2. Place the cream cheese in the center of the plastic wrap, and then add another layer of plastic wrap on top.

3. Using a rolling pin, roll the cream cheese until it is even and about 1/4 inch thick.

4. Try to make the shape somewhat resemble a rectangle.

5. Pull off the top layer of plastic wrap.

6. Place the salami slices so they overlap to cover the cream-cheese layer completely.

7. Place a new piece of plastic wrap on top of the salami layer to flip over your cream cheese–salami rectangle. Flip the layer, so the cream cheese side is up.

8. Remove the plastic wrap and add the sliced pepperoncini in a layer on top.

9. Roll the layered ingredients into a tight log, pressing the meat and cream cheese together. (You want it as tight as possible.)

10. Then wrap the roll with plastic wrap and refrigerate for at least 6 hours so it will set.

11. Slice and serve.

Nutrition: Calories: 141 Fat: 4.9g Fiber: 2.1g Carbohydrates: 0.3 g Protein: 8.5g

35. Zucchini Balls with Capers and Bacon

Preparation Time: 3 hrs.

Cooking Time: 20 minutes

Servings: 10

Ingredients:

- 2 zucchinis, shredded
- 2 bacon slices, chopped
- 1/2 cup cream cheese, at room temperature
- 1cup fontina cheese
- 1/4 cup capers
- 1 clove garlic, crushed
- 1/2 cup grated Parmesan cheese
- 1/2 tsp. poppy seeds
- 1/4 tsp. dried dill weed
- 1/2 tsp. onion powder
- Salt and black pepper, to taste
- 1 cup crushed pork rinds

Directions:

1. Preheat oven to 360 F.
2. Thoroughly mix zucchinis, capers, 1/2 of Parmesan cheese, garlic, cream cheese, bacon, and fontina cheese until well combined.
3. Shape the mixture into balls.

4. Refrigerate for 3 hours.

5. In a mixing bowl, mix the remaining Parmesan cheese, crushed pork rinds, dill, black pepper, onion powder, poppy seeds, and salt.

6. Roll cheese ball in Parmesan mixture to coat.

7. Arrange in a greased baking dish in a single layer and bake in the oven for 15-20 minutes, shaking once.

Nutrition: Calories: 227 Fat: 12.5g Fiber: 9.4g Carbohydrates: 4.3 g Protein: 14.5g

36. Strawberry Fat Bombs

Preparation Time: 30 minutes

Cooking Time: 0 minutes

Servings: 6

Ingredients:

- 100 g strawberries
- 100 g cream cheese
- 50 g butter
- 2 tbsp. erythritol powder
- 1/2 teaspoon vanilla extract

Directions:

1. Put the cream cheese and butter (cut into small pieces) in a mixing bowl.
2. Let rest for 30 to 60 minutes at room temperature.
3. In the meantime, wash the strawberries and remove the green parts.
4. Pour into a bowl and process into a puree with a serving of oil or a mixer.
5. Add erythritol powder and vanilla extract and mix well.
6. Mix the strawberries with the other ingredients and make sure that they have reached room temperature.
7. Put the cream cheese and butter into a container.

8. Mix with a hand mixer or a food processor to a homogeneous mass.

9. Pour the mixture into small silicone muffin molds. Freeze.

Nutrition: Calories: 95 Fat: 9.1g Fiber: 4.1g Carbohydrates: 0.9 g Protein: 2.1g

37. Plantains with Tapioca Pearls

Preparation Time: 15 Minutes

Cooking Time: 3 Hours

Servings: 6

Ingredients:

- 5ripe plantains, sliced into thick disks
- 1can thick coconut cream
- 1tsp. coconut oil
- 1/4cup tiny tapioca pearls, dried
- 1cup white sugar
- 2cups water
- Pinch of salt

Directions:

1. Grease the Instant Pot Pressure Cooker with coconut oil.

2. Place ripe plantains. Top this with tapioca pearls, coconut oil, white sugar, and salt. Pour just the right amount of water into the Instant Pot.

3. Lock the lid in place. Press the high pressure and cook for 5 minutes.

4. When the beep sounds, Choose the Quick Pressure Release. This will depressurize for 7 minutes. Remove the lid.

5. Tip in in coconut cream. Allow residual heat cook the last ingredient.

6. To serve, ladle just the right amount of plantains into dessert bowls.

Nutrition: Calories 345 Fat 8 Fiber 4.5 Carbs 3.5 Protein 20

VEGETABLES RECIPES

38. Gouda Cauliflower Casserole

Preparation Time: 15 minutes

Cooking Time: 15 minutes

Servings: 4

Ingredients:

- 2 heads cauliflower, cut into florets
- 1/3 cup butter, cubed
- 2 tbsp. melted butter
- 1white onion, chopped
- Salt and black pepper to taste
- 1/4 almond milk
- 1/2 cup almond flour
- 1 1/2 cups grated gouda cheese

Directions:

1. Preheat oven to 350ºF and put the cauliflower florets in a large microwave-safe bowl.

2. Sprinkle with a bit of water, and steam in the microwave for 4 to 5 minutes.

3. Melt the 1/3 cup of butter in a saucepan over medium heat and sauté the onion for 3 minutes.

4. Add the cauliflower, season with salt and black pepper, and mix in almond milk. Simmer for 3 minutes.

5. Mix the remaining melted butter with almond flour.

6. Stir into the cauliflower as well as half of the cheese. Sprinkle the top with the remaining cheese and bake for 10 minutes until the cheese has melted and golden brown.

7. Plate the bake and serve with salad.

Nutrition: Calories: 349 Fat: 9.4g Fiber: 12.1g Carbohydrates: 4.1 g Protein: 10g

39. Spinach and Zucchini Lasagna

Preparation Time: 15 minutes

Cooking Time: 30 minutes

Servings: 4

Ingredients:

- 2 zucchinis, sliced
- Salt and black pepper to taste
- 2 cups ricotta cheese
- 2 cups shredded mozzarella cheese
- 3 cups tomato sauce
- 1cup baby spinach

Directions:

1. Let the oven heat to 375 and grease a baking dish with cooking spray.

2. Put the zucchini slices in a colander and sprinkle with salt.

3. Let sit and drain liquid for 5 minutes and pat dry with paper towels.

4. Mix the ricotta, mozzarella cheese, salt, and black pepper to evenly combine and spread 1/4 cup of the mixture in the bottom of the baking dish.

5. Layer 1/3 of the zucchini slices on top spread 1 cup of tomato sauce over, and scatter a 1/3 cup of spinach on top. Repeat process.

6. Grease one end of foil with cooking spray and cover the baking dish with the foil.

7. Let it bake for about 35 minutes. And bake further for 5 to 10 minutes or until the cheese has a nice golden-brown color.

8. Remove the dish, sit for 5 minutes, make slices of the lasagna, and serve warm.

Nutrition: Calories: 376 Fat: 14.1g Fiber: 11.3g Carbohydrates: 2.1 g Protein: 9.5g

40. Lemon Cauliflower "Couscous" with Halloumi

Preparation Time: 5 minutes

Cooking Time: 5 minutes

Servings: 2

Ingredients:

- 4 oz halloumi, sliced
- cauliflower head, cut into small florets
- 1/4 cup chopped cilantro
- 1/4 cup chopped parsley
- 1/4 cup chopped mint
- 1/2 lemon juiced
- Salt and black pepper to taste
- Sliced avocado to garnish

Directions:

1. Heat the pan and add oil
2. Add the halloumi and fry on both sides until golden brown, set aside. Turn the heat off.
3. Next, pour the cauliflower florets in a food processor and pulse until it crumbles and resembles couscous.
4. Transfer to a bowl and steam in the microwave for 2 minutes.
5. They should be slightly cooked but crunchy.

6. Stir in the cilantro, parsley, mint, lemon juice, salt, and black pepper.

7. Garnish the couscous with avocado slices and serve with grilled halloumi and vegetable sauce.

Nutrition: Calories: 312 Fat: 9.4g Fiber: 11.9g Carbohydrates: 1.2 g Protein: 8.5g

POULTRY RECIPES

41. Cheesy Roasted Chicken

Preparation Time: 15 minutes

Cooking Time: 10 minutes

Servings: 6

Ingredients:

- 3 cups of chopped roasted chicken
- 2cups of shredded cheddar cheese
- 2cups white of shredded cheddar cheese
- 3 cups of shredded parmesan cheese

Directions:

1. Oven: 350F
2. Be sure to rub butter or to spray with non-stick cooking spray.
3. In a bowl, put in all the cheese and mix well.
4. Microwave the cheese till it melts
5. Put in the chicken and toss thoroughly.
6. Put two tablespoons of the cheese chicken combo in a pile on the baking sheet. Be sure to leave space between piles.
7. Bake for 4-6 minutes. The moment they turn golden brown at the edges, take them off.

8. Serve hot.

Nutrition: Calories: 387 Fat: 19.5g Fiber: 4.1g Carbohydrates: 3.9 g Protein: 14.5g

42. Spiced Duck Goulash

Preparation time: 15 minutes

Cooking time: 5 minutes

Servings: 2

Ingredients:

- 2(1-ounce / 28-g) slices bacon, chopped
- ½ pound (227 g) duck legs, skinless and boneless
- 2cups chicken broth, preferably homemade
- ½ cup celery ribs, chopped
- 2green garlic stalks, chopped
- 2green onion stalks, chopped
- 1ripe tomato, puréed
- Kosher salt, to season
- ¼ teaspoon red pepper flakes
- ½ teaspoon Hungarian paprika
- ½ teaspoon ground black pepper
- ½ teaspoon mustard seeds
- ½ teaspoon sage
- 1bay laurel

Directions:

1. Heat a stockpot over medium-high heat; once hot, fry the bacon until it is crisp or about 3 minutes. Add in the duck legs and cook until they are no longer pink.

2. Chop the meat, discarding any remaining skin and bones. Then, reserve the bacon and meat.

3. Pour in a splash of chicken broth to deglaze the pan.

4. Now, sauté the celery, green garlic and onions for 2to 3 minutes, stirring periodically. Add the remaining ingredients to the pot, including the reserved bacon and meat.

5. Stir to combine and reduce the heat to medium-low. Let it cook, covered, until everything is thoroughly heated or about 1hour. Serve in individual bowls and enjoy!

Nutrition: calories: 364 fats: 22.4g protein: 33.2g carbs: 5.1g net carbs: 3.7g fiber: 1.4g

43. Chicken Spinach Salad

Preparation Time: 15 minutes

Cooking Time: 0 minutes

Servings: 3

Ingredients:

- 21/2cups of spinach
- 4 1/2ounces of boiled chicken
- 2boiled eggs
- 1/2cup of chopped cucumber
- 3 slices of bacon
- 1small avocado
- 1tablespoon olive oil
- 1/2teaspoon of coconut oil
- Pinch of Salt
- Pepper

Directions:

1. Dice the boiled eggs.
2. Slice boiled chicken, bacon, avocado, spinach, cucumber, and combine them in a bowl. Then add diced boiled eggs.
3. Drizzle with some oil. Mix well.
4. Add salt and pepper to taste.
5. Enjoy.

Nutrition: Calories: 265 Fat: 9.5g Fiber: 10.5g Carbohydrates: 3.3 g Protein: 14.1g

44. Thai Peanut Chicken Skewers

Preparation Time: 10 minutes

Cooking Time: 15 minutes

Servings: 2

Ingredients:

- 1-pound boneless skinless chicken breast, cut into chunks
- 3 tablespoons coconut aminos
- 1/2teaspoon Sriracha sauce, plus 1/4 teaspoon
- 3 teaspoons toasted sesame oil, divided
- Ghee, for oiling
- 2tablespoons peanut butter
- Pink Himalayan salt
- Freshly ground black pepper

Directions:

1. In a bag, combine the chicken chunks with two tablespoons of soy sauce, 1/2teaspoon of Sriracha sauce, and two teaspoons of sesame oil. Marinate the chicken.

2. If you are using wood 8-inch skewers, soak them in water for 30 minutes before using.

3. Oil the grill pan with ghee.

4. Thread the chicken chunks onto the skewers.

5. Cook the skewers over low heat for 10 to 15 minutes, flipping halfway through.

6. Meanwhile, mix the peanut dipping sauce.

7. Stir together the remaining one tablespoon of soy sauce, 1/4 teaspoon of Sriracha sauce, one teaspoon of sesame oil, and the peanut butter.

8. Season with pink Himalayan salt and pepper.

9. Serve the chicken skewers with a small dish of the peanut sauce.

Nutrition: Calories: 390 Fat: 18.4 g Fiber: 12.9g Carbohydrates: 2.1g Protein: 17.4g

FISH AND SEAFOOD RECIPES

45. Bacon and Feta Skewers

Preparation Time: 15 minutes

Cooking Time: 10 minutes

Servings: 4

Ingredients:

- 2lb. feta cheese, cut into 8 cubes
- 8 bacon slices
- 4 bamboo skewers, soaked
- 1zucchini, cut into 8 bite-size cubes
- Salt and black pepper to taste
- 3 tbsp. almond oil for brushing

Directions:

1. Wrap each feta cube with a bacon slice.
2. Thread one wrapped feta on a skewer; add a zucchini cube, then another wrapped feta, and another zucchini.
3. Repeat the threading process with the remaining skewers.
4. Preheat a grill pan to medium heat, generously brush with the avocado oil and grill the skewer on both sides for 3 to 4 minutes per side or until the set is golden brown and the bacon cooked.

5. Serve afterward with the tomato salsa.

Nutrition: Calories: 290 Fat: 15.1g Fiber: 4.2g Carbohydrates: 4.1g Protein: 11.8g

46. Avocado and Prosciutto Deviled Eggs

Preparation Time: 20 minutes

Cooking Time: 10 minutes

Servings: 4

Ingredients:

- 4 eggs
- Ice bath
- 4 prosciutto slices, chopped
- 1avocado, pitted and peeled
- 1tbsp. mustard
- 1tsp. plain vinegar
- 1tbsp. heavy cream
- 1tbsp. chopped fresh cilantro
- Salt and black pepper to taste
- 1/2cup (113 g) mayonnaise
- 1tbsp. coconut cream
- 1/4 tsp. cayenne pepper
- 1tbsp. avocado oil
- 1tbsp. chopped fresh parsley

Directions:

1. Boil the eggs for 8 minutes.
2. Remove the eggs into the ice bath, sit for 3 minutes, and then peel the eggs.

3. Slice the eggs lengthwise into halves and empty the egg yolks into a bowl.

4. Arrange the egg whites on a plate with the hole side facing upwards.

5. While the eggs are cooked, heat a non-stick skillet over medium heat and cook the prosciutto for 5 to 8 minutes.

6. Remove the prosciutto onto a paper towel-lined plate to drain grease.

7. Put the avocado slices to the egg yolks and mash both ingredients with a fork until smooth.

8. Mix in the mustard, vinegar, heavy cream, cilantro, salt, and black pepper until well-blended.

9. Spoon the mixture into a piping bag and press the mixture into the egg holes until well-filled.

10. In a bowl, whisk the mayonnaise, coconut cream, cayenne pepper, and avocado oil.

11. On serving plates, spoon some of the mayonnaise sauce and slightly smear it in a circular movement. Top with the deviled eggs, scatter the prosciutto on top and garnish with the parsley.

12. Enjoy immediately.

Nutrition: Calories: 265 Fat: 11.7g Fiber: 4.1g Carbohydrates: 3.1g Protein: 7.9 g

47. Artichoke and Avocado Pasta Salad

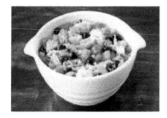

Preparation Time: 15 minutes

Cooking Time: 30 minutes

Servings: 10 Servings:

Ingredients:

- Two cups of spiral pasta (uncooked)
- A quarter cup of Romano cheese (grated)
- One can (fourteen oz.) of artichoke hearts (coarsely chopped and drained well)
- One avocado (medium-sized, ripe, cubed)
- Two plum tomatoes (chopped coarsely)
- For the dressing:
- One tablespoon. of fresh cilantro (chopped)
- Two tablespoons. of lime juice
- A quarter cup of canola oil
- One and a half teaspoons. of lime zest (grated)
- Half a teaspoon. each of

- Pepper (freshly ground)
- Kosher salt

Directions:

1. Follow the directions mentioned on the package for cooking the pasta. Drain them well and rinse using cold water.

2. Then, take a large-sized bowl and in it, add the pasta along with the tomatoes, artichoke hearts, cheese, and avocado. Combine them well. Then, take another bowl and add all the ingredients of the dressing in it. Whisk them together and, once combined, add the dressing over the pasta.

3. Gently toss the mixture to coat everything evenly in the dressing and then refrigerate.

Nutrition: Calories: 188 Protein: 6g Fat: 10g Carbs: 21g Fiber: 2g

48. Apple Arugula and Turkey Salad in a Jar

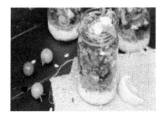

Preparation Time: 10 minutes

Cooking Time: 10 minutes

Servings: 4 Servings:

Ingredients:

- Three tablespoons. of red wine vinegar
- Two tablespoons. of chives (freshly minced)
- Half a cup of orange juice
- One to three tablespoons. of sesame oil
- A quarter teaspoon. each of
- Pepper (coarsely ground)
- Salt
- For the salad:
- Four teaspoons. of curry powder
- Four cups each of
- Turkey (cubed, cooked)
- Baby spinach or fresh arugula
- A quarter teaspoon. of salt

- Half a teaspoon. of pepper (coarsely ground)
- One cup of halved green grapes
- One apple (large-sized, chopped)
- Eleven oz. of mandarin oranges (properly drained)
- One tablespoon. of lemon juice
- Half a cup each of
- Walnuts (chopped)
- Dried cranberries or pomegranate seeds

Directions:

1. Take a small-sized bowl and, in it, add the first 6 ingredients from the list into it. Whisk them. Then take a large bowl and in it, add the turkey and then add the seasonings on top of it. Toss the turkey cubes to coat them with the seasoning. Take another bowl and in it, add the lemon juice and toss the apple chunks in the juice.

2. Take four jars and divide the layers in the order I mention here - first goes the orange juice mixture, the second layer is that of the turkey, then apple, oranges, grapes, cranberries or pomegranate seeds, walnuts, and spinach or arugula. Cover the jars and then refrigerate them.

Nutrition: Calories: 471 Protein: 45g Fat: 19g Carbs: 33g Fiber: 5g

DESSERT

49. Chocolate Mousse

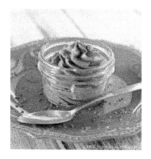

Preparation Time: 15 Minutes

Cooking Time: 3 Hours

Servings: 6

Ingredients:

- 16 ounces' cream cheese
- 3-6 tablespoons of desired sweetener
- 1/2cup unsweetened cocoa powder
- 1/2cup heavy whipped cream
- 1large avocado
- 90% dark chocolate, to garnish
- 1/4 teaspoon vanilla extract

Directions:

1. Beat cream cheese until it becomes smooth and creamy, slowly mix cocoa powder.

2. Add avocado and beat it nicely for 5 minutes until it becomes creamy.

3. Add vanilla and sweetener, and then beat it again until it becomes creamy and smooth.

4. Place the whipped cream in the chocolate mixture and fold gently. Place the chocolate mousse in the desired containers. Garnish with dark chocolate chips.

Nutrition: Calories 345 Fat 8 Fiber 4.5 Carbs 3.5 Protein 20

50. Salted Vanilla Caramels

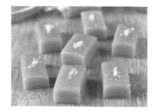

Preparation time: 5 minutes

Cooking time: 15 minutes

Servings: 24

Ingredients:

- 2tablespoons unsalted butter, at room temperature
- 1cup all lose
- ¼ teaspoon sea salt
- ¼ cup heavy whipping cream
- ½ teaspoon vanilla extract

Directions:

1. Line the baking pan with wax paper and set aside.

2. In a small saucepan, brown the butter over medium heat for about 3 minutes, making sure to stir often while the butter browns. Add the all lose and stir until well combined. Simmer for about 7 minutes, until melted, then stir in the salt. Once it starts to bubble, add the heavy cream and vanilla and stir constantly, making sure it doesn't boil over. Once combined, reduce the heat and allow to gently simmer for about 3 minutes, until reduced slightly.

3. Remove the caramel sauce from the heat and pour it evenly into the prepared baking pan. Put into the refrigerator for a couple of hours or overnight, until cool and hardened.

4. Cut the caramel into 24 pieces and serve.

5. To store, wrap each candy in wax paper, twisting the sides closed. Put the candies in an airtight container in the refrigerator for up to 5 days. With refrigeration, the candies will become very firm but will soften at room temperature.

Nutrition: calories: 5 fat: 0.8g protein: 0g carbs: 0g net carbs: 0g fiber: 0g

CONCLUSION

The ketogenic diet is a great way to lose weight quickly and improve your overall health. However, it can be difficult to stick with the keto diet when eating out, and snacking on the wrong foods makes it hard for you to get back on track. The key is to pack your own food or find restaurants where it's possible to order low carb dishes like grilled fish, vegetable salads, or chicken breast with green vegetables and avocado.

The keto diet is a nutritional lifestyle that helps you lose weight and manage your blood sugar levels. If you follow the ketogenic diet, you must reduce carbohydrates to no more than ten percent of your total daily calories. Carbs in foods like breads, pastas, rice, and beans will have a negative impact on your weight loss. And avoid limiting your carbs when you go out to eat. The following tips will help you pack a healthy meal on the go while still being able to stick to your keto diet.

Choose wisely when choosing your carbohydrate sources. For example, avoid bread and pasta in large portions as they provide empty calories without providing any good nutrients. Instead, choose fruit, vegetables, meat, or seafood instead of processed foods that are loaded with empty calories and will contribute to your weight gain.

If you're dining out at a fast food restaurant, bring along low carb snacks that offer good nutrition and taste great – but are also low in carbs. This will prevent you from overeating.

If you do not have low carb pasta alternatives, you could try grilled chicken and vegetables with pesto sauce. That way you're getting healthy greens without carbs.

Lightning Source UK Ltd.
Milton Keynes UK
UKHW022016190421
382278UK00003B/615